PHARMACIST (DR) FRANCIS SAMUEL

PAPILLOMAVIRUS Effects and management

Contents

Acknowledgement

My acknowledgement goes to those who dedicated their time in sharing and contributing towards the success of this book through; typing of the manuscript painstakingly, financial assistance and previewing the manuscript. I really appreciate ..thanks

Chapter One

INTRODUCTION

Papilloma virus (HPV) is a kind of virus which mostly affect the skin and the mucus membranes, often times most of these viruses are not easily detected because most of them do not show a health issues for a long period of time while some are death trap because of their deadly action on skin and membranes. HPV are know to possess a cancer threat on its host and thereby damages tissue more easily if left untreated.

Human papillomavirus has been diagnosed in both men and women all over the world and there are more than 200 types of HPV across the globe. Because of the mostly asymptomatic nature of these viruses, their transmission become more rapid and undetectable from different individuals and can be spread through sex (including vaginal, oral, anal sex), body contact. It is most paramount that young adults and adult who are sexually active to at least check their status from time to time because early detection matters a lot in managing HPV. Some of the issues associated with HPV includes: warts, cervical cancer mouth infection and others.

Chapter Two

TYPES AND VARIANTS

The human papillomavirus, or HPV, has been found in more than 200 distinct forms and kinds. These may be roughly divided among two primary groups according to their possible health consequences and risk variables such as;

2.1 RELATIVELY SAFE TYPES OF HPV:

Highest warts on the genitals are caused by HPV types 6 and 11, which are the most prevalent relatively safe type of HPV types. In broad terms, there is a lower likelihood of major health issues arising from them.

2.2 EXTREMELY SUSCEPTIBLE TYPES OF HPV:

HPV 16 and 18: Due to their substantial correlation with the emergence of several infections, including cervical cancer, these two forms of the virus are the most alarming. Extremely susceptible HPV strains have the potential to cause the throat and other genital cancers

2.3. OTHER EXTREMELY SUSCEPTIBLE TYPES:

A number of extremely susceptible HPV types, including 31, 33, 45, 52, and 58, are associated with an increased risk of cancer in together with HPV 16 and 18.

It's critical to remember that not every kind of HPV has the same threats to health. While genital warts can be caused by some relatively harmless varieties, these are not usually linked to disease. Conversely, extremely susceptible varieties increase the chance of developing cancer in the mouth, vulva, cervix, anus, penis, and vagina.

Vaccines, including the HPV vaccination, provide safeguards against some of the greatest number of harmful forms of HPV by targeting certain types of HPV that are highly hazardous. Comprehending the many forms and variants of HPV is essential for averting health hazards, identifying them early, and managing them. Immunizations and periodic examinations are useful preventative measures in decreasing the problem of extremely susceptible HPV variants

Chapter Three

TRANSMISSION:

1. SEXUAL INTERACTION: Vaginal, anal, and oral sex are among the main ways that HPV is spread. When the virus gets into touch with the salivary glands of the mouth, anal, or genitalia, it can spread. Sexual practices that are penetrative or not can transmit an infection.

2. SKIN-TO-SKIN CONTACT: Non-sexual skin-to-skin contact is another way that HPV can spread. This implies that there is a chance of infection even in locations that are not protected by a condom. For example, the virus can spread through hand-genital touch.

3. DIRECT TRANSFER: In rare circumstances, an infected mother may pass on HPV to her infant after childbirth, which might cause the kid to develop genital or respiratory infections.

3.2. INFECTION RISK FACTORS:
   The following variables may make an HPV infection more likely:

1. SEXUAL ENGAGEMENT: The risk of HPV contamination and transmission is higher in those who have several sexual partners or who engage in sexual activities when they are younger.

2. ABSENCE OF VACCINATION: HPV vaccination, which guards against some potentially hazardous types, might increase the risk of infection, particularly in younger people.

3. POOR IMMUNE SYSTEM: People who use medicines that suppress immunity or have illnesses like HIV may have a weaker immune system, which increases their susceptibility to HPV and its repercussions.

4. GENITAL WARTS: The danger of contracting or spreading additional HPV strains is elevated in individuals with genital warts, that are brought on by minimal-risk HPV kinds.

5. TOBACCO USE: Smoking increases the chance of HPV infection-related cervical cancer.

6. GENDER: Although HPV affects both men and women, specific viruses can cause cancer of the cervix in women, among other more serious side effects.

Knowing how HPV spreads and what makes people more susceptible to infection is essential if you want to lower your risk of infection by obtaining frequent examinations, being vaccinated against HPV, and using secure sexual methods.

Chapter Four

RELATED DISEASES:

HPV can cause a number of health problems, from common warts to more serious illnesses, especially some forms of cancer. These are a few of the main illnesses linked to HPV:

1. CERVICAL CANCER.

Constant infection with highly susceptible HPV types, particularly HPV 16 and 18, increases the risk of cervical cancerous cell growth. For the purposes of early identification and mitigation, routine HPV screening and Pap smear examinations are crucial.

2. OTHER GENITAL CANCERS:

In addition to the vulva, vagina, anus, and penis, HPV can also result in cancer in these other genital regions. Although less frequent than cervical cancer, these tumors are linked to highly susceptible HPV strains.

3. THE THROAT CANCER:

Certain HPV strains, especially HPV 16, have the ability to infect the mouth and throat, which can result in cancers of the mouth These cancers have been more common than

4. GENITAL WARTS:

The development of genital warts is caused by moderately risky HPV types, including HPV 6 and 11. These warts can develop in the mouth, throat, and anal region in addition to the genitalia. They may need to be treated even though they are not deadly. They can be irritating.

Rarely, HPV can result in respiratory papillomatosis, a condition in which warts develop in the trachea and larynx, among other airways. This may cause breathing problems and need to be surgically removed.

Knowing the connection between HPV and these illnesses emphasizes how crucial early identification and avoidance are. Secure sexual habits, periodic checks, and HPV vaccination are essential for lowering the risk of HPV-related illnesses, especially cancer.

4.1 CERVICAL CANCER:

One kind of cancer that starts in the cervix—the lower portion of the uterus that joins the vagina—is called cervical cancer. It is one of the greatest prevalent cancers that affect women globally and is closely associated with extremely susceptible HPV strains, specifically HPV 16 and 18. Here include a few essential details regarding cervical cancer:

CAUSES: Cervical cancer is primarily caused by persistent infection with high-risk HPV types. Cervical cells can become infected with HPV, which may ultimately result in precancerous and malignant cells to grow.

SYMPTOMS: Cervical cancer may not exhibit any signs in its initial phases. However, as the cancer worsens, symptoms like irregular vaginal bleeding, pelvic pain, pain during sexual activity, and strange vaginal discharge may appear.

SCREENING AND PREVENTION: To detect precancerous changes in the cervix early, routine screenings are necessary. Examples of these screenings include Pap smears and HPV tests. Another very successful routine method against the most prevalent types with the greatest risk of is the HPV vaccine.

TREATMENT: Depending on the disease's stage, there are various treatment options for cervical cancer. These could consist of chemotherapy, radiation therapy, surgery, or a mix of these. The woman's age, general
health, and cancer stage all influence the treatment plan that is

chosen.

PROGNOSIS: Cervical cancer can have an extensive number of outcomes, but it is typically treatable if caught promptly and handled. For cervical cancer that is specific, the 5-year survival rate is comparatively high. But as the cancer progresses, the prognosis gets worse.

IMPACT AND PREVALENCE: Cervical cancer is still a major public health concern, particularly in places where screening initiatives and healthcare are scarce. In order to lessen the incidence of cervical cancer, regular tests and immunization campaigns are essential.

PREVENTION: The best ways to prevent and detect cervical cancer are to have safe sexual behavior, get the HPV vaccine (which is typically advised for people before they start having sexual relations), and have regular screenings for the disease.

Cervical cancer might be prevented and treated, and lowering death rates and enhancing outcomes are largely dependent on early identification via tests.

4.2 GENITAL WARTS

Condylomata acuminata, another name for genital warts, are a common sexually transmitted infection (STI) that is mainly caused by moderately risky strains of the Human Papillomavirus (HPV), such as HPV 6 and 11. Here are a number of essential details regarding vaginal warts:

CAUSES: HPV 6 and 11 are the main causes of genital warts. These variants of HPV can cause warts to develop by infecting the skin and mucous membranes of the genital and anal regions.

LOOK: Small, flesh-colored or gray growths or lumps on or near the genitalia or anal region constitute the typical form of genital warts. They can be raised, flat, or shaped like cauliflowers, depending on their size.

SYMPTOMS: Although vaginal warts rarely cause any symptoms or discomfort, they can occasionally itch, hurt, or bleed. Sometimes they can be seen with the unaided eye, and other times they might be internal and difficult to find without a medical examination.

TRANSMISSION: Vaginal, anal, and oral sex are among the sexual contacts that can result in the spread of genital warts, which are extremely contagious. Even in cases where there are no visible warts, they can still spread through skin-to-skin contact.

TREATMENT: Topical drugs, cryotherapy (freezing), laser therapy, or surgical excision are available for the treatment of vaginal warts. Seeking advice from a medical expert is crucial for the right diagnosis and course of treatment.

RECURRENCE: Because the virus may stay dormant in the body, genital warts may recur even after successful treatment. It is imperative to schedule routine follow-ups with a healthcare professional in order to monitor and manage any recurrences.

PREVENTION: The risk of genital warts can be decreased by vaccination against certain
high-risk and low-risk HPV types. Use of condoms and other safe sexual practices can also aid in the prevention of transmission.

Although genital warts are usually not linked to cancer, they can cause both physical and psychological discomfort. Genital warts can be managed and their negative effects on a person's health and well-being can be minimized with early diagnosis and appropriate treatment.

4.3 OTHER CANCERS ASSOCIATED BY HPV

Human Papillomavirus, or HPV, is linked to multiple cancer types in addition to cervical cancer. These cancers can arise as a result of high-risk HPV strains, particularly HPV 16 and 18. These additional cancers have been connected to HPV:

4.3.1 CANCER OF THE OROPHARYNX: This kind of cancer affects the tonsils, base of the tongue, and throat. Oropharyngeal cancer is significantly increased by HPV, especially HPV-16. Oropharyngeal cancer linked to HPV has been more common in recent years, particularly in younger people.

4.3.2 ANAL CANCER: Anal cancer has been linked to HPV. It has the potential to infect the anal lining and cause cancerous cells to grow. Individuals with compromised immune systems and those with a history of anal warts are more vulnerable to anal cancer.

4.3.3 VAGINAL CANCER: HPV can cause vaginal cancer, though this is comparatively uncommon. Most cases of HPV are caused by high-risk strains. Early detection is aided by routine Pap tests and gynecological exams.

4.3.4 VULVAR CANCER: Another uncommon but dangerous cancer connected to HPV infection is vulvar cancer. It happens on the external genital region. Vulvar cancer is linked to the emergence of high-risk HPV strains.

4.3.5 PENILE CANCER: HPV is associated with a higher risk of developing penile cancer, especially when high-risk HPV types are present. Frequent medical examinations and self-examinations can aid in early detection.

4.3.6 RARER CANCERS: HPV has also been linked to less frequent cancers, including skin, throat, and mouth cancers. The particular HPV strains involved in these cases may differ.

The best way to lower the risk of these HPV-associated cancers is through prevention, such as HPV vaccination and responsible sexual behavior. The likelihood that affected people will receive effective treatment and recover from their condition can be increased by early detection through screenings and quick medical attention.

Chapter Five

SYMPTOMS AND DIAGNOSIS OF HPV

5.1 SYMPTOMS:

GENITAL WARTS: A few HPV strains, particularly low-risk varieties like HPV 6 and 11, have the potential to cause genital warts. Small, flesh-colored growths on or near the genital and anal regions may be the appearance of these warts.

No Symptoms: HPV infections frequently have no outwardly visible symptoms. It is possible for people to carry the virus unknowingly and not get sick.

5.2 DIAGNOSIS:

1. CLINICAL EXAMINATION: A medical professional can frequently diagnose vaginal warts caused by HPV through a visual examination.

2. PAP SMEAR: Pap smears, also known as Pap tests, are used on cervixes to identify changes in cervical cells brought on by HPV. Additional testing might be necessary if abnormal cells are discovered.

3. HPV TEST: HPV testing can determine whether cervical cells contain high-risk HPV strains. This test is frequently run either alone or in combination with a Pap smear.

4. BIOPSY: To confirm the existence of abnormalities related to HPV or cervical cancer, a biopsy may be carried out if there are suspicious growths

or lesions.

5. ORAL AND OROPHARYNGEAL HPV: A biopsy or imaging tests are usually required for the diagnosis of HPV-related cancers of the mouth and throat, including oropharyngeal cancer.

It's crucial to remember that although clinical exams and testing can identify HPV and the problems it causes, the virus may not always be found. Furthermore, there isn't a standard HPV test for other body parts.

Regular screenings are essential for early detection of HPV-related health issues, particularly cervical cancer. For some high-risk HPV types, vaccination against HPV is also an effective preventive measure.

Chapter six

VACCINATION

Vaccination against the human papillomavirus (HPV) is a highly effective method of protection against certain strains of the virus, particularly the low-risk strains that cause genital warts and the high-risk strains that can cause cancer. Important details about HPV vaccination are as follows:

1. VACCINE: Currently available HPV vaccines are Cervarix and Gardasil 9. Gardasil 9, one of the most widely used, protects against nine different types of HPV, including those that are responsible for the majority of anal, cervical, and oropharyngeal cancers.

2. TARGET POPULATION FOR VACCINE: HPV vaccinations are recommended prior to sexual activity, which is typically around age 11 or 12. However, older individuals who have not had a vaccination can also get one.

3. DOSAGE SCHEDULE: Multiple injections are required to administer the HPV vaccine. Depending on the age and type of vaccination, the schedule for doses may vary. It is usually necessary to take two or three doses spaced out over several months.

4. CERVICAL CANCER PREVENTION: Vaccination against HPV has been shown to significantly reduce the risk of cervical cancer by targeting high-risk HPV types. It also provides protection against other related malignancies, such as oropharyngeal and anal cancers.

5. PREVENTION OF GENITAL WARTS: Vaccinations also offer protection

against low-risk HPV types that can cause genital warts.

6. EFFECTIVENESS: HPV vaccinations significantly improve the prevention of HPV infections, which can lead to serious health issues. However, they are most effective when taken before engaging in sexual activity that could expose you to the virus.

7. SAFETY: HPV vaccinations are regarded to be safe and rarely cause serious side effects. Common side effects include fever, lightheadedness, and soreness or swelling where the injection was made.

8. IMPACT ON THE WORLD: Worldwide vaccination campaigns against HPV have the capacity to significantly reduce the incidence of diseases and cancers associated with HPV.

HPV vaccination is an essential public health measure for preventing diseases linked to HPV, particularly cervical cancer. In order to maximize the benefits of immunizations, parents, guardians, and medical professionals need to understand their importance and follow recommended schedules.

Chapter Seven

SAFE PRACTICES AND PREVENTION OF HPV AND RELATED DISEASES

Vaccination and safe practices are two ways to prevent human papillomavirus (HPV) and the illnesses it causes. The following are important precautions:

1. THE HPV VACCINE:

Before engaging in any sexual activity, teenagers should usually be vaccinated against HPV, which may protect against both low- and high-risk strains of the virus. These vaccinations are quite successful in lowering the risk of illnesses linked to HPV, such as genital warts and cervical cancer.

2. APPROPRIATE SEXUAL BEHAVIOR:

Although they may not provide total protection, condoms can help lower the risk of HPV transmission when used appropriately and regularly. This is because the virus can still infect places that the condom does not cover.

The risk of HPV exposure may be decreased by cutting down on the number of sexual partners.

Selecting a monogamous sexual partner who is not afflicted might also lessen the chance of HPV transmission.

3. FREQUENT EXAMS:

Frequent screenings are necessary for the early diagnosis of abnormalities in cervical cells and other HPV-related problems. These screenings include Pap smears and HPV testing.

4. STEER CLEAR OF SMOKE:

For those infected with HPV, smoking is linked to an increased risk of cervical cancer. Reducing your smoking may reduce this risk.

5. AWARENESS ABOUT HPV:

Having knowledge about HPV, how it spreads, and the illnesses it may cause is essential for making well-informed choices on healthcare and prevention.

6. SECURE ORAL SEXUAL BEHAVIORS:

Using condoms or dental dams may lower the risk of HPV transmission for oral sex partners, especially for oropharyngeal HPV.

7. EDUCATION ON HPV:

Young people may be encouraged to be vaccinated before engaging in sexual activity by being educated about HPV and the value of vaccination.

8. FREQUENT MEDICAL EXAMS:

Frequent checkups with the doctor may aid in the early diagnosis of HPV-related disorders, such as genital warts and certain malignancies.

Reducing the effects of HPV and related disorders requires prevention. Safe sexual behaviors and HPV vaccination are essential elements of these initiatives. Healthcare professionals and public health initiatives are essential in raising awareness and encouraging vaccination to shield people from HPV-related illnesses.

Chapter Eight

TREATMENT OPTIONS FOR HPV

It's crucial to remember that although there is no known cure for the Human Papillomavirus (HPV), there are treatments for the potential health problems it might bring. The following are the available treatments for HPV-related conditions:

8.1 MEDICINE FOR GENITAL WARTS:

1 TOPICAL MEDICATIONS: Genital warts may be treated with prescription creams or solutions to help get rid of them. Usually, these procedures are carried out at home.

2. CRYOTHERAPY A standard in-office technique involves freezing the warts with liquid nitrogen.

Surgery: Warts that are resistant to conventional therapies may need to be surgically removed.

Changes in Cervical Cells and Cervical Cancer:

3. CERVICAL DYSPLASIA: Treatment may be required if precancerous abnormalities in the cervix are found. Procedures such as conization (cone biopsy), LEEP (loop electrosurgical excision technique), or cryotherapy may be used in this.

Cervical disease: Depending on the stage and extent of the disease, treatment options for cervical cancer may include surgery, radiation therapy, chemotherapy, or a combination of these.

Other HPV-related malignancies such as those of the anal, oropharyngeal, vaginal, vulvar, or penile regions may be treated with immunotherapy, chemotherapy, radiation treatment, or targeted therapies. The kind and stage of the cancer determines the precise treatment approach.

4. INHALATIONAL PAPILLOMATOSIS:

Surgical Excision: To remove papillomas (warts) from the airway in patients with recurrent respiratory papillomatosis (RRP), surgery is often necessary. Over time, it could be necessary to repeat these steps.

5. FREQUENT OBSERVATION:

In order to assess development and provide prompt intervention if required, careful monitoring by a healthcare practitioner is essential for many HPV-related illnesses, including precancerous alterations.

It's critical to stress that addressing HPV-related health concerns requires early identification and swift medical action. One of the most important methods for lowering the prevalence of these disorders is prevention, which includes safe sexual behavior and HPV vaccination. See a healthcare professional for advice and the best care if you think you may have an HPV-related problem or have concerns about treatment.

Chapter Nine

FREQUENTLY ASKED QUESTION (FAQs)

Of course! Frequently asked questions (FAQs) about the human papillomavirus (HPV) are included below:

1. DESCRIBE HPV.

A family of viruses known as HPV, or human papillomavirus, affects the skin and mucous membranes. Certain varieties may result in health problems, such as vaginal warts and certain forms of cancer.

2. HOW DOES HPV SPREAD?

The main way that HPV is spread is via sexual contact, which includes oral, anal, and vaginal intercourse. Additionally, non-sexual skin-to-skin contact might transmit it.

3. WHAT HPV SYMPTOMS ARE PRESENT?

Many HPV carriers may not show any symptoms. When signs do appear, they might include warts on the genitalia, abnormal Pap screen findings, or, in more severe situations, cancer-related symptoms.

4. IS HPV CURABLE?

While HPV cannot be cured, the majority of infections do. Treatment is available for HPV-related illnesses such cervical cell alterations and genital warts.

5. HOW MAY MALIGNANCIES LINKED TO HPV BE AVOIDED?

One important line of defense against certain high-risk HPV strains linked to cancer is HPV vaccination. Preventive measures also include refraining from tobacco usage, healthy sexual behavior, and routine checkups.

6. WHEN IS THE RIGHT AGE TO GET THE HPV VACCINE?

Adolescents should have the HPV vaccination, preferably before they start having sex, which is usually around the ages of 11 or 12. It may, however, be given up until age 26.

7. DOES THE HPV VACCINATION WORK?

It is true that the HPV vaccination works very well to protect against infections caused by the majority of high-risk and low-risk HPV strains. It offers robust defense against genital warts and cervical cancer.

8. ARE MALES SUSCEPTIBLE TO HPV?

Indeed, guys may get HPV. They may get anal cancer, genital warts, and other illnesses linked to HPV. For men, the HPV vaccination is also advised.

9. HOW FREQUENTLY SHOULD PAP TESTS BE PERFORMED ON WOMEN?

Pap smear frequency is influenced by a number of variables, including age, medical history, and HPV vaccination status. Routine tests typically begin at age 21 and are carried out every three to five years.

10. CAN NON-SEXUAL INTERACTION RESULT IN THE TRANSMISSION OF HPV?

It is true that non-sexual skin-to-skin contact may transfer HPV, even though sexual transmission is the predominant method of viral transmission.

These responses only cover broad topics; for more tailored guidance, those with particular questions or medical issues should speak with medical specialists.